Galactosemia Cookbook For Kids

Delicious and Safe Recipes for Children with Galactosemia

Justine C COLE

<u>DISCLAIMER.</u>

As fellow advocates for those battling galactosemia, we understand the daily challenges and emotional toll this condition can take. This cookbook is crafted with utmost care and empathy, with the hope of providing not just nourishment, but also comfort and support on your journey. Each recipe is thoughtfully designed to be galactosemia-friendly, with ingredients that prioritise your health and well-being. While we strive for accuracy and safety, we urge you to consult with your healthcare provider before making any dietary changes. Your health and happiness are our top priorities, and we stand with you every step of the way."

DEDICATION

"To the brave souls navigating the challenges of Galactosemia,

In the face of adversity, you shine with unmatched strength and resilience. This cookbook is dedicated to you—warriors who bravely confront each day with unwavering determination and courage.

May these pages serve as a reminder of your indomitable spirit and unwavering perseverance. You are not defined by your condition, but by the remarkable fortitude with which you face it.

In every recipe lies a testament to your unwavering resolve, a celebration of your triumphs, both big and small. You are not alone on this journey; you are surrounded by a community of warriors who understand, support, and uplift each other.

Through every meal prepared with love and care, may you find nourishment for both body and soul. Your strength inspires us all, and your resilience knows no bounds.

With heartfelt admiration and endless support,

JUSTINE C COLE

Table of Contents

CHAPTER:8 BEYOND THE KITCHEN
8.1.LIVING WELL WITH GALACTOSEMIA.

Conclusion

BONUS PAGE.

WHY THIS BOOK

*T*he "Galactosemia Cookbook" penned by Justine C. Cole isn't just any ordinary cookbook—it's a culinary guide tailored specifically for those navigating the complexities of galactosemia. With years of culinary expertise under my belt, I can confidently say that this book is a vital resource for anyone seeking flavorful yet galactosemia-friendly dishes.

From the moment you crack open the spine, you're immersed in a culinary journey that goes beyond the basics. The initial chapters serve as a comprehensive introduction to galactosemia, providing clear insights into its nuances. But it doesn't stop there—armed with knowledge, you're empowered to manage galactosemia with confidence.

Now, onto the heart of the book—chapters filled with over 100 meticulously crafted recipes. These dishes are not only delicious but also tailored to accommodate galactosemia restrictions. From satisfying breakfast options to decadent desserts, each recipe showcases the fusion of taste and functionality, inspiring endless culinary possibilities.

And there's more! Alongside the recipes, you'll find bonuses like a 30-day meal plan, ensuring mealtime is stress-free and nutritious. Plus, insider tips and kitchen gadget recommendations enhance your culinary journey.

With the "Galactosemia Cookbook" by your side, you can bid farewell to the confusion of online searches and conflicting advice. This book is your trusted companion, offering a roadmap to culinary success while prioritising your health and well-being.

So, whether you're a kitchen novice or a seasoned chef, this book promises something special for everyone. Dive in and explore on a culinary adventure that will tantalise your taste buds and support your health journey.

How to Use This Book

1.Get Acquainted: Start by flipping through the introductory chapters to familiarise yourself with galactosemia and its dietary implications. This foundational knowledge sets the stage for your journey.

2.Explore the Recipes: Over 100 thoughtfully curated recipes await, spanning from breakfast to dessert. Each dish is expertly crafted to be both delicious and galactosemia-friendly, ensuring that every meal is a delight.

3.Plan Your Meals: Take advantage of the included 30-day meal plan for hassle-free meal planning. This comprehensive guide ensures that your meals are not only nutritious but also varied and satisfying.

4.Cook with Confidence: Armed with insider tips and kitchen gadget recommendations sprinkled throughout the book, approach each recipe with assurance. Whether you're a kitchen novice or a seasoned chef, you'll find everything you need to create masterpieces.

5.Embrace Variety: Experiment with different recipes and flavour combinations to keep your meals exciting. With a plethora of options at your fingertips, you'll never run out of inspiration.

6.Prioritize Your Health: Rest assured that each recipe is meticulously crafted to adhere to galactosemia restrictions while prioritising flavour and nutrition. With the "Galactosemia Cookbook," you can enjoy delicious meals without compromising your health.

<u>**7.Share the Joy:**</u> Spread the love by sharing your creations with friends and family. Whether it's a cosy family dinner or a festive gathering, let the flavours of the "Galactosemia Cookbook" bring people together.

INTRODUCTION

*W*elcome to the "Galactosemia Cookbook for Kids." As a seasoned chef, I've always believed that food should not only nourish our bodies but also bring joy and comfort to our lives. This book is especially close to my heart because it addresses a unique and often challenging dietary need with creativity, warmth, and love. Whether you're a parent, caregiver, or a young reader living with galactosemia, this cookbook is designed to bring delicious, safe, and fun meals to your table.

Imagine being nine years old and discovering that the food you love can make you sick. This was Jennie's reality. A bright and lively girl, Jennie was diagnosed with galactosemia at a young age. For those who may not be familiar, galactosemia is a rare genetic disorder that affects the body's ability to process galactose, a sugar found in milk and many other foods. This means that even a small amount of dairy can cause serious health problems for someone like Jennie.

Jennie's early years were filled with unexplained pains and discomforts. Her parents, not knowing the cause, were helpless and heartbroken seeing their little girl suffer. After countless doctor visits and tests, Jennie was diagnosed with galactosemia. While the diagnosis brought relief in knowing the cause, it also ushered in a new set of challenges. The family had to completely overhaul their diet, cutting out all forms of dairy and many other foods that contained hidden sources of galactose.

The initial transition was tough. Jennie missed her favourite foods—ice cream, cheese pizza, and even simple treats like cookies and milk. Her parents struggled to find suitable replacements that were both safe and enjoyable. Meals became a source of stress rather than joy. They often found themselves in the kitchen, experimenting with different ingredients, trying to create dishes that Jennie could eat without risking her health. It was a daunting task that felt overwhelming at times.

Then, something wonderful happened. Jennie's family stumbled upon a cookbook specifically designed for children with galactosemia. It was like a light at the end of a long, dark tunnel. For the first time, they had a resource filled with recipes that were safe, delicious, and fun to make. The cookbook transformed their kitchen from a place of frustration to a place of creativity and joy. Jennie loved getting involved in the cooking process, turning it into a family activity. Together, they discovered new favourite dishes, adapted old ones, and found a sense of normalcy and happiness in their meals once again.

This "Galactosemia Cookbook for Kids" is inspired by stories like Jennie's. It's crafted with care to provide a comprehensive guide for families navigating the complexities of a galactosemia-friendly diet. Here, you'll find an array of recipes that cater to the needs of children with galactosemia without compromising on taste or fun. From breakfast to dinner, snacks to desserts, each recipe is carefully designed to be easy to follow, nutritionally balanced, and most importantly, enjoyable for kids.

The benefits of this cookbook extend far beyond just providing recipes. It aims to educate and empower families, helping them understand galactosemia better and manage it with confidence. You'll learn about safe ingredients, how to read food labels, and tips for dining out. The cookbook also includes personal stories and tips from other families living with galactosemia, offering a sense of community and support.

Cooking for a child with galactosemia doesn't have to be a chore. This book is filled with vibrant, flavorful recipes that kids will love, making mealtime a joyful experience. Whether it's crafting a delicious dairy-free mac and cheese, whipping up a batch of cookies, or preparing a hearty, comforting soup, this cookbook turns challenges into opportunities for creativity and bonding.

Jennie's story is just one among many, but it encapsulates the struggles and triumphs that come with managing galactosemia. Through the pages of this cookbook, I hope to bring a sense of hope, normalcy, and delight to your kitchen. Cooking is an art, but it's also a way to connect with those we love. By using this cookbook, you're not just making meals—you're creating memories, building a supportive community, and ensuring that children with galactosemia can enjoy the same joys of food and family that everyone else does.

In the United States, where food culture is rich and diverse, having a resource like this is invaluable. It allows families to partake in traditional and contemporary American cuisines without the worry of galactose-related complications. From classic American dishes to innovative new favorites, this cookbook ensures that children with galactosemia can enjoy a varied and fulfilling culinary experience.

This cookbook is more than a collection of recipes; it's a beacon of hope and a celebration of resilience. As you turn the pages and try out the recipes, remember Jennie's journey and know that you're not alone. There are many families out there who understand your challenges and are cheering you on. Together, we can transform mealtime into a source of joy, comfort, and endless delicious possibilities.

Chapter:1 UNDERSTANDING GALACTOSEMIA

WHAT IS GALACTOSEMIA?

Galactosemia is a condition where the body can't handle a sugar called galactose, found in foods like dairy. If untreated, it can lead to liver issues, cataracts, speech difficulties, and mental impairment.

HOW COMMON IS GALACTOSEMIA?

"Galactosemia, a genetic disorder, affects about 1 in every 30,000 babies. A milder form called the Duarte variant is more common, affecting around 1 in 16,000 newborns."

WHAT GENES ARE RELATED TO GALACTOSEMIA?.

Most cases of galactosemia come from mutations in genes. These mutations affect enzymes needed to process galactose, a sugar found in many foods.

- ***Type I galactosemia has two forms:*** classic and Duarte variant. In the classic type, there's very little enzyme activity to process galactose. In the Duarte variant, there's some enzyme activity, but not enough to cause symptoms.
- ***Type II galactosemia is caused*** by mutations in the GALK1 gene, leading to a shortage of the enzyme galactokinase.

- *Type III galactosemia is due* to mutations in the GALE gene, causing a shortage of the enzyme UDP-galactose-4-epimerase. These enzymes are also important for galactose metabolism.

HOW DO PEOPLE INHERIT GALACTOSEMIA?

This condition is passed down when both parents carry a changed gene, but they usually don't show symptoms themselves. For someone to have the disorder, they need to inherit two altered genes, one from each parent.

WHAT IS THE NORMAL FUNCTION OF THE GALE GENE?

The GALE gene gives instructions for making an enzyme called UDP-galactose-4-epimerase. This enzyme helps our bodies process the sugar galactose, found in dairy. It converts sugars like UDP-galactose to UDP-glucose, which cells use for energy and building fats and proteins.

WHAT CONDITIONS ARE RELATED TO THE GALE GENE?

Galactosemia - Caused by Mutations in the GALE Gene

There are two types of UDP-galactose-4-epimerase deficiency, called galactosemia type III, which are caused by changes in the GALE gene. These types are known as mild (peripheral) and severe (generalised) deficiency.

TYPES OF GALACTOSEMIA?

Galactosemia, a rare genetic disorder, manifests in various types, each presenting unique challenges and symptoms. Understanding these types is crucial for accurate diagnosis and tailored treatment plans.

1.Classic Galactosemia:
This type results from mutations in the GALT gene, leading to deficient enzyme activity. Infants with classic galactosemia often display symptoms shortly after birth, including jaundice, liver enlargement, and failure to thrive. If left untreated, it can lead to severe complications such as intellectual disability and cataracts.

2.Duarte Galactosemia: Unlike classic galactosemia, individuals with Duarte galactosemia have partial enzyme activity, typically around 25-50% of normal levels. While symptoms may be milder compared to classic galactosemia, affected individuals still need careful monitoring and dietary restrictions to prevent complications.

3.Galactokinase Deficiency: This type results from mutations in the GALK1 gene, affecting the galactokinase enzyme responsible for converting galactose to galactose-1-phosphate. Infants with galactokinase deficiency may develop cataracts in early infancy if galactose intake is not controlled. However, unlike classic galactosemia, intellectual development is usually unaffected.

4.Epimerase Deficiency Galactosemia: This rare form stems from mutations in the GALE gene, impairing the function of the epimerase enzyme. Individuals with this type may experience similar symptoms to classic galactosemia, including liver dysfunction and developmental delays. However, the severity of symptoms can vary widely among affected individuals.

5.UDP-Galactose-4-Epimerase Deficiency:
Also known as Type III galactosemia, this type is extremely rare and results from mutations in the GALE gene, similar to epimerase deficiency galactosemia. Symptoms may include developmental delays, liver dysfunction, and cataracts, but more research is needed to fully understand its clinical presentation and management.

SYMPTOMS AND DIAGNOSIS

Galactosemia is a rare genetic issue where the body can't handle galactose, a sugar in milk. Babies with this condition might struggle to feed, vomit, or have diarrhea. If not treated, it can lead to serious problems like liver damage, eye issues, and learning difficulties. Doctors use tests to diagnose it early. Treatment involves avoiding foods with galactose and lactose, like dairy products. Regular check-ups are important to monitor growth and prevent problems. It's crucial for medical professionals to spot and manage galactosemia properly to help those affected live well.

Chapter:2

HUMAN ENZYMES UNDERLYING GALACTOSEMIA

This project aims to understand how genetic mutations affect enzymes involved in galactose metabolism, which is crucial for preventing galactosemia, a serious genetic disorder. By studying two key enzymes, GALT and GALE, and their mutations, we hope to uncover why some mutations cause more severe problems than others. Our short-term goals include understanding the structures and functions of these enzymes and how they influence metabolism and glycosylation in cells. This research could lead to better diagnosis, prognosis, and treatment options for galactosemia patients.

Chapter:3

ALTERNATIVE MEDICINE AND GALACTOSEMIA

As medical practitioners and culinary experts, we understand the profound impact of dietary interventions and alternative medicine on managing genetic disorders like galactosemia. Galactosemia, a metabolic disorder affecting approximately 1 in 114,000 live births, demands a comprehensive approach that integrates conventional medical treatments with alternative modalities, including dietary modifications and herbal remedies.

From a medical perspective, galactosemia presents unique challenges due to its biochemical and clinical heterogeneity. Traditional medical treatments often focus on enzyme replacement therapy and dietary restrictions to mitigate the adverse effects of galactose accumulation in the body. However, alternative medicine offers a complementary avenue for addressing the underlying metabolic imbalances and promoting holistic well-being.

Herbal remedies, such as dandelion root and milk thistle, have shown promising results in supporting liver function and aiding in the detoxification process, which is crucial for individuals with galactosemia who experience liver complications. Additionally, acupuncture and acupressure can help alleviate symptoms associated with galactosemia, such as fatigue and gastrointestinal distress, by restoring the body's energy flow and promoting relaxation.

From a culinary perspective, dietary modifications play a pivotal role in managing galactosemia and optimizing overall health outcomes. As seasoned professional chefs, we recognize the importance of creating delicious and nutritious meals that adhere to the dietary restrictions imposed by galactosemia. By focusing on fresh, whole foods and incorporating alternative ingredients such as coconut milk and almond flour, we can craft innovative dishes that cater to individuals with galactosemia while satisfying their taste buds.

Furthermore, fermenting foods rich in galactose, such as dairy products, can help break down lactose into more easily digestible components, thereby reducing the risk of galactose accumulation in the body. Fermented foods like yoghourt and kefir not only provide beneficial probiotics but also offer a flavorful alternative to traditional dairy products.

Incorporating nutrient-dense ingredients like leafy greens, legumes, and lean proteins into meal plans can help meet the nutritional needs of individuals with galactosemia while promoting optimal health and vitality. By emphasising variety and balance in our culinary creations, we can ensure that individuals with galactosemia receive the essential nutrients they need to thrive.

In conclusion, the integration of alternative medicine approaches and culinary expertise holds tremendous promise for enhancing the management of galactosemia. By embracing holistic interventions that address the biochemical complexities of the disorder and nourish the body with wholesome, flavorful foods, we can empower individuals with galactosemia to lead fulfilling and vibrant lives. As advocates for holistic health and culinary creativity, we remain committed to exploring innovative strategies that promote well-being and resilience in the face of genetic challenges like galactosemia.

Galactose-Free Pantry Essentials

1.Non-Dairy Milk Alternatives: One of the first swaps you'll need to make in your galactose-free pantry is replacing dairy milk with non-dairy alternatives. Stock up on options like almond milk, coconut milk, soy milk, or oat milk. These alternatives provide the creamy texture and richness you crave without the galactose found in traditional cow's milk. Use them in everything from cereal and coffee to baking and cooking savoury sauces.

2.Plant-Based Butter: Butter adds richness and flavour to countless recipes, but it's a no-go for those avoiding galactose. Luckily, there are plenty of plant-based butter options available that deliver the same delicious results. Look for varieties made from ingredients like coconut oil, avocado oil, or olive oil. These alternatives can be used in baking, sautéing, and spreading on toast with confidence.

3.Nutritional Yeast: Nutritional yeast is a versatile ingredient that adds a cheesy, umami flavour to dishes without any dairy products. It's a must-have in any galactose-free pantry for creating cheesy sauces, seasoning popcorn, or sprinkling over roasted vegetables. Nutritional yeast is also packed with essential vitamins and minerals, making it a nutritious addition to your meals.

4.Coconut Cream: For creamy soups, sauces, and desserts, coconut cream is a lifesaver in the galactose-free kitchen. This rich and indulgent ingredient adds depth of flavour and luxurious texture to a variety of dishes. Use it to thicken curries, whip up dairy-free whipped cream, or create decadent desserts like coconut cream pie or dairy-free ice cream.

5.Alternative Flours: Traditional wheat flour contains gluten and may not be suitable for those with galactose intolerance. Thankfully, there are plenty of alternative flours available that are both gluten-free and galactose-free. Stock your pantry with options like almond flour, coconut flour, rice flour, or chickpea flour. These flours can be used in baking, breading, and thickening sauces, providing a nutritious and delicious alternative to wheat flour.

6.Agar Agar: Agar agar is a natural gelling agent derived from seaweed, making it a perfect substitute for gelatin in galactose-free recipes. Use agar agar to set desserts like panna cotta or jelly without relying on dairy-based ingredients. It's also a great way to thicken sauces and soups without adding any galactose-containing dairy products.

7. Coconut Aminos: If you're looking to add depth of flavour to your dishes without using soy sauce, coconut aminos are a fantastic alternative. Made from the sap of coconut blossoms, coconut aminos have a similar savoury taste to soy sauce without the soy or galactose. Use them in marinades, stir-fries, dressings, or as a dipping sauce for sushi and spring rolls.

Substitutes for Dairy Products

When it comes to cooking, dairy products can play a starring role in many dishes, adding richness, creaminess, and flavour. However, for those who are lactose intolerant, allergic to dairy, or following a vegan lifestyle, finding suitable substitutes can be a game-changer. As a seasoned professional chef, I've explored various alternatives to dairy products, and I'm here to share my insights to help you navigate this culinary landscape.

Let's start with milk. Traditional cow's milk can be easily replaced with plant-based alternatives such as almond milk, soy milk, oat milk, or coconut milk. Each of these options offers its own unique flavour profile and consistency, allowing you to choose the best one for your recipe. Almond milk, for example, adds a subtle nuttiness, while coconut milk brings a hint of tropical sweetness.

Next up, let's talk about cheese. While nothing quite replicates the exact taste and texture of cheese made from cow's milk, there are several dairy-free options that come pretty close. Look for plant-based cheeses made from ingredients like nuts, soy, or tapioca starch. These cheeses melt beautifully and can be used in everything from sandwiches to pasta dishes to cheese boards. Experiment with different brands and varieties to find the ones you like best.

Butter is another essential dairy product that can easily be swapped out. Margarine made from plant oils is a popular choice, but there are also dairy-free butter alternatives made from ingredients like coconut oil or avocado oil. These alternatives can be used in baking, sautéing, or simply spread on toast for a dairy-free delight.

When it comes to creamy sauces and dressings, coconut cream is a fantastic substitute for heavy cream. Its rich texture and subtle sweetness make it perfect for everything from curries to desserts. Simply chill a can of coconut milk overnight, then scoop out the thick cream that rises to the top. Whisk it until smooth, and you've got yourself a dairy-free cream alternative that's sure to impress.

Yoghurt lovers need not despair, as there are plenty of dairy-free options available. Look for yoghourts made from coconut milk, almond milk, or soy milk, which offer the same tangy flavour and creamy texture as traditional yoghurt. These dairy-free yoghurts are perfect for enjoying on their own, or you can use them in smoothies, parfaits, or as a topping for granola.

Finally, let's not forget about ice cream. While dairy-free ice cream may have once been a rarity, it's now widely available in grocery stores and specialty shops. Made from ingredients like coconut milk, almond milk, or soy milk, these frozen treats come in a variety of flavours and are every bit as creamy and delicious as their dairy counterparts.

Hidden Sources of Galactose

Today, I'm excited to share with you a revelation that many overlook: the hidden sources of galactose. Galactose is a lesser-known sugar, often overshadowed by its more famous counterpart, glucose. But understanding where it hides in our foods is crucial for both culinary excellence and health-conscious cooking.

Let's start with dairy products. Milk, cheese, and yoghurt are well-known sources of galactose, as it is a component of lactose, the sugar naturally present in dairy. But did you know that even lactose-free dairy products can contain galactose? During the process of making lactose-free dairy, enzymes break down lactose into its component sugars, including galactose. So, if you're aiming to reduce galactose intake, it's essential to read labels carefully and opt for truly lactose-free alternatives.

Moving beyond dairy, another surprising source of galactose is legumes. Beans, lentils, and chickpeas contain a type of carbohydrate called galactooligosaccharides, or GOS, which our bodies break down into galactose during digestion. While legumes are undoubtedly nutritious and a staple in many cuisines, those seeking to limit galactose intake may want to moderate their consumption.

Next on our list are fruits and vegetables. While most fruits contain primarily fructose, the sugar found in fruits like apples, pears, and grapes also contains a small amount of galactose. Similarly, certain vegetables, such as Brussels sprouts, contain naturally occurring galactose. While these foods offer numerous health benefits, individuals following a low-galactose diet may need to be mindful of their intake.

Another unexpected source of galactose is certain grains. Grains like wheat, barley, and oats contain a carbohydrate known as galactan, which our bodies metabolise into galactose. While whole grains are an essential part of a balanced diet, those seeking to reduce galactose intake may opt for alternative grains such as quinoa or rice.

Finally, let's not forget about hidden sources of galactose in processed foods. Many packaged snacks, desserts, and sauces contain ingredients derived from dairy, legumes, or grains, which can contribute to galactose intake. Reading ingredient labels and choosing whole, minimally processed foods whenever possible is key to minimising galactose consumption.

In Summary , while galactose may be a lesser-known sugar, its presence in our food is significant. As a seasoned professional chef, I urge you to consider the hidden sources of galactose when crafting your culinary creations. By being mindful of ingredients and making informed choices, you can ensure that your dishes are both delicious and aligned with your nutritional goals. So, next time you step into the kitchen, remember to keep an eye out for galactose and unleash the full potential of your cooking prowess.

Shopping Tips for a Galactose-Free Diet

When navigating the aisles for a galactose-free diet, it's all about mastering the art of label reading and understanding which foods are safe to indulge in and which ones to steer clear of. As a seasoned professional chef who has been crafting delicious dishes for years, I've picked up some invaluable tips along the way that I'm excited to share with you.

First and foremost, let's talk about what galactose is and why it matters. Galactose is a type of sugar found in dairy products and some other foods. For individuals with galactosemia, a condition where the body cannot properly metabolise galactose, consuming foods containing this sugar can lead to serious health issues. That's why it's crucial to be diligent when it comes to food choices.

When hitting the grocery store, always start by checking the ingredients list on packaged foods. Look out for sneaky sources of galactose, such as milk, cheese, yoghourt, and butter. These ingredients should send up a red flag and prompt you to put the item back on the shelf. Instead, opt for dairy-free alternatives like almond milk, coconut yoghourt, and vegan cheese.

But it's not just dairy products you need to be wary of. Galactose can also hide in unexpected places, like certain breads, cereals, and processed foods. Ingredients such as whey, casein, lactose, and lactulose are all indicators that a product contains galactose and should be avoided.

Fresh fruits and vegetables are your best friends when following a galactose-free diet. Not only are they naturally free from galactose, but they also provide essential nutrients and fibre to keep you feeling satisfied and energised. Get creative in the kitchen by incorporating a variety of colourful produce into your meals, from crunchy carrots and leafy greens to juicy berries and sweet potatoes.

When it comes to protein sources, there are plenty of galactose-free options to choose from. Lean meats like chicken, turkey, and fish are safe bets, as are plant-based proteins like tofu, tempeh, and legumes. Just be sure to double-check any pre-marinated or processed meats for hidden sources of galactose.

Grains can be a bit trickier to navigate, but fear not! Stick to gluten-free options like rice, quinoa, and oats to avoid any potential sources of galactose. Whole grains are not only nutritious but also versatile, making them perfect for everything from hearty salads to comforting porridge.

When in doubt, remember that fresh is best. By focusing on whole, unprocessed foods and cooking from scratch whenever possible, you can take control of your diet and ensure that every bite is galactose-free and bursting with flavour. With a little bit of planning and a whole lot of creativity, eating galactose-free can be not only manageable but downright delicious. So go ahead, hit the kitchen, and let your culinary imagination run wild!

COOKING WITH KIDS

SAFETY IN THE KITCHEN

I've seen how vital it is to ensure the safety and well-being of every child we cook for, especially those with specific dietary needs like galactosemia. Galactosemia is a condition where the body can't process galactose, a sugar found in milk and dairy products. This means our kitchen practices need to be not only meticulous but also mindful of avoiding any harmful ingredients. Here are some key safety tips and guidelines to follow when cooking for kids with galactosemia.

Kitchen Cleanliness

Start with a clean kitchen. Ensure all surfaces, utensils, and cooking equipment are thoroughly cleaned before you begin. Cross-contamination can occur easily, so it's essential to use separate cutting boards, knives, and pots for galactose-free cooking. Wash your hands frequently and ensure all ingredients are clearly labelled and stored separately.

Ingredient Awareness

Read labels carefully. Many processed foods contain hidden sources of galactose. Ingredients like casein, whey, lactose, and milk solids must be avoided. Opt for fresh, whole foods whenever possible, and choose plant-based alternatives like almond milk, coconut milk, and soy products that do not contain galactose. However, always double-check labels for any added ingredients that might be harmful.

Safe Substitutions

Learn to substitute safely. In place of dairy, use plant-based milks and cheeses. For baking, you can use applesauce or mashed bananas as a replacement for butter. Nutritional yeast can add a cheesy flavor to dishes without any dairy. Explore these alternatives to create dishes that are both safe and tasty for children with galactosemia.

Meal Planning

Plan meals that are naturally free of dairy. Think about incorporating a variety of fruits, vegetables, grains, and proteins that don't require substitution. For example, a stir-fry with tofu, colourful vegetables, and rice is a great option. Salads with a variety of toppings, grilled meats, and hearty soups made with vegetable broth are also safe and nutritious choices.

Cooking Techniques

Master simple cooking techniques that enhance flavours without relying on dairy. Roasting vegetables brings out their natural sweetness, while grilling adds a smoky depth to meats and vegetables. Use herbs and spices to add flavour and complexity to your dishes. These techniques can make a big difference in the taste and appeal of your meals.

Educating Others

If you're cooking in a household or setting where others are involved, educate them about galactosemia and the importance of strict dietary adherence. Make sure everyone understands the need to avoid cross-contamination and to read labels carefully. Create a supportive environment where everyone works together to ensure the safety of the child with galactosemia.

Note:

Cooking for kids with galactosemia requires attention to detail, but with the right knowledge and practices, you can create safe and delicious meals. Always stay vigilant about ingredient labels, maintain a clean kitchen, and embrace the use of fresh, whole foods. By doing so, you'll not only ensure their safety but also introduce them to a world of flavours and nutritious options. Cooking with care and creativity can make every meal enjoyable and safe for kids with galactosemia.

FUN COOKING ACTIVITIES

Cooking for kids with galactosemia requires creativity, knowledge, and a lot of fun. I've discovered many engaging activities that not only help in managing this condition but also make cooking an exciting adventure for kids.

Galactosemia means avoiding foods that contain galactose, a sugar found in milk and dairy products. But don't worry—there are plenty of ways to keep meals delicious and nutritious.

Here are some enjoyable cooking activities tailored for children with galactosemia.

1.Exploring Fruits and Vegetables:
Kids love exploring new things, and what better way than with fruits and vegetables? Let them pick out different kinds of produce at the grocery store or farmers' market. Talk about the colours, shapes, and textures. When you get home, you can make fun fruit and veggie faces on their plates. This activity not only teaches them about healthy eating but also makes mealtime fun.

2. DIY Salad Bar:
Set up a DIY salad bar at home. Provide a variety of safe ingredients like leafy greens, carrots, cucumbers, tomatoes, and beans. Let the kids create their own salads. They can mix and match different items and experiment with flavours. This helps them learn about making healthy choices and gives them a sense of independence.

3.Smoothie Creations:
Smoothies are a great way to pack in nutrients. Kids can choose their favourite fruits and veggies to blend. Use a base of almond milk or any other non-dairy milk. Add some fun extras like chia seeds, spinach, or berries. Let the kids press the buttons on the blender (with supervision, of course). They'll love seeing their ingredients transform into a tasty drink.

4.Homemade Popsicles:
Making popsicles is a fantastic way to cool down and have fun. Use fruit juices and purees. Kids can help pour the mixtures into moulds. You can even add in small pieces of fruit for extra texture. Freeze them, and in a few hours, you have a delicious, galactose-free treat.

5.Fun with Baking:

Baking is a wonderful way to introduce kids to cooking. There are many recipes that can be adapted to be galactose-free. Use non-dairy alternatives like coconut oil and almond milk. Let the kids help measure ingredients, mix batter, and decorate the baked goods. This activity not only teaches them about cooking but also about patience and following instructions.

6.Creative Sandwiches:

Making sandwiches can be a fun and artistic activity. Use whole grain bread and let the kids choose from a variety of fillings like turkey, chicken, hummus, and lots of veggies. Use cookie cutters to make fun shapes. This makes lunchtime exciting and gives them control over what they eat.

7 Build Your Own Pizza:

Pizza night can be transformed into a fun cooking activity. Use a galactose-free crust and let the kids add their toppings. Provide options like tomato sauce, veggies, grilled chicken, and non-dairy cheese. They can get creative with their toppings and make faces or patterns. It's a fun way to get them involved in cooking.

8.Fun with Herbs and Spices:

Introduce kids to different herbs and spices. Let them smell and taste each one. Talk about how these can be used to flavour food. You can even plant a small herb garden together. This teaches them about where food comes from and adds an educational element to cooking.

9.Making Healthy Snacks:

Involve kids in making their own snacks. You can make trail mix with nuts, seeds, and dried fruits. Let them mix the ingredients themselves. This way, they can have a snack that's both healthy and fun to make.

10.Cooking Competitions:

Organise a friendly cooking competition at home. Give the kids a few ingredients and let them come up with their own dishes. Judge them on creativity and taste. This can be a great way to encourage their cooking skills and make them feel like little chefs.

Cooking for kids with galactosemia doesn't have to be boring. With these fun activities, you can turn the kitchen into a playground of learning and creativity. It's all about making food exciting and safe. These activities not only help manage their dietary needs but also foster a love for cooking that can last a lifetime.

Chapter:4

Breakfast Delights

---

1. Spinach Feta Egg Wrap

Prep Time:10 mins

Cook Time:5 mins

Total Time:15 mins

Servings:1

Ingredients

- 1 large whole-wheat tortilla
- 1 ½ teaspoons coconut oil
- 1 cup chopped baby spinach leaves
- 1 oil-packed sun-dried tomato, chopped
- 2 eggs, beaten
- ⅓ cup feta cheese
- 1 tomato, diced

Directions

1. Heat a tortilla in a large skillet over medium heat.

2. In another skillet, melt coconut oil over medium-high heat. Cook spinach and tomato until spinach wilts, about 1 minute. Add eggs and scramble for about 2 minutes until almost set. Sprinkle feta cheese on top and cook for another minute until it melts.

3. Place the scrambled egg mixture on the warm tortilla; add diced tomato on top. Roll the tortilla and heat in the skillet for about 30 seconds until it holds its shape.

<u>**Nutritional value**</u>

Carbs=81g

Protein=40g

Calories=705

Fat=39g

2.Carnation Chocolate Raspberry Breakfast Parfait

Prep Time:10 mins

Total Time:10 mins

Servings:2

Ingredients

- 1 Packet CARNATION BREAKFAST ESSENTIALS Rich Milk Chocolate Powdered Drink Mix
- 1 (5.3 ounce) container plain Greek yoghourt
- ¼ cup graham cracker crumbs
- ¼ cup fresh raspberries
- 1 (5.3 ounce) container raspberry Greek yoghourt

Directions

1. Stir chocolate drink mix into plain Greek yogurt until well combined.

2. In two parfait glasses, layer 2 1/2 tablespoons of the chocolate yogurt mixture, 2 teaspoons of graham cracker crumbs, some raspberries, and 2 1/2 tablespoons of raspberry yogurt. Repeat the layers to finish the parfaits.

<u>Nutritional value</u>

Carbs=31g

Protein=12g

Calories=247

Fat=9g

3.Avocado Toast and Egg for One

Prep Time:10 mins

Cook Time:10 mins

Total Time:20 mins

Servings:1

Ingredients

- 1 small shallot, thinly sliced into rings
- 1 tablespoon red wine vinegar
- salt to taste
- 1 small avocado, pitted and peeled
- ¼ lime, juiced
- 1 egg
- 1 tablespoon white vinegar
- freshly ground black pepper to taste
- 1 slice whole-grain crusty bread
- 1 pinch Aleppo pepper, to taste

Directions

1. Mix shallot, red wine vinegar, and a pinch of salt in a bowl; set aside. In another bowl, mash avocado with lime juice and salt.

2. Bring 2 to 3 inches of water to a boil in a shallow saucepan. Add vinegar and reduce to a simmer. Crack an egg into a ramekin and gently slide it into the simmering water. Poach for 3 to 4 minutes until the white is set and the yolk is soft. Remove with a slotted spoon and place on a paper towel-lined plate. Season with salt and pepper.

3. Toast bread and place it on a plate. Top with mashed avocado, some pickled shallot, and the poached egg. Sprinkle with Aleppo pepper and serve immediately.

Nutritional value

Carbs=35g
Protein=14g
Calories=478
Fat=31g

4.Strawberry-Banana Freezer Oatmeal.

Prep Time:10 mins

Cook Time:5 mins

Additional Time:8 hrs 10 mins

Total Time:8 hrs 25 mins

Servings:18

Ingredients

- 1 cup white sugar, divided
- 2 cups fresh strawberries, sliced
- 3 cups water
- 2 cups almond milk
- 2 ½ cups old-fashioned oats
- 1 ½ cups bananas, mashed
- 1 teaspoon cinnamon
- 1 teaspoon vanilla extract
- ¼ teaspoon salt
- ⅛ teaspoon ground nutmeg
- ½ cup pecans, chopped

Directions

1. Sprinkle 1/2 cup of sugar over sliced strawberries in a bowl and let sit for 10 to 15 minutes until juices are released.

2. In a large pot, boil water and almond milk. Add oats and cook on medium-low for 5 minutes, stirring often. Mix in strawberries, remaining 1/2 cup of sugar, bananas, cinnamon, vanilla extract, salt, and nutmeg, then remove from heat. Stir in pecans.

3. Grease 18 muffin cups and fill each with the oat mixture, slightly mounding the tops. Freeze for 8 hours or overnight. Remove the frozen oatmeal from the muffin cups and store in freezer bags or a freezer-safe container.

4. To prepare, microwave a frozen oatmeal cup in a microwave-safe bowl for 1 1/2 to 2 minutes.

<u>Nutritional value</u>
Carbs=26g
Protein=2g
Calories=141
Fat=3g

5.Justine C Cole Whole Grain Pancakes

Prep Time:15 mins

Cook Time:20 mins

Total Time:35 mins

Servings:28

Ingredients

- 1 cup all-purpose flour
- 1 ⅓ cups dry milk powder
- 1 teaspoon baking powder
- 1 ½ teaspoons baking soda
- 1 teaspoon salt
- 2 cups whole wheat flour
- ¾ cup white sugar
- 4 eggs, lightly beaten
- 3 cups water
- ¼ cup butter, melted
- 3 tablespoons vinegar

Directions

1. In a large bowl, sift together all-purpose flour, milk powder, baking powder, baking soda, and salt. Stir in whole wheat flour. In a small bowl, mix sugar, eggs, water, butter, and vinegar. Make a well in the flour mixture and pour in the egg mixture. Mix until smooth.

2. Heat a lightly oiled griddle or frying pan over medium heat. Pour about 1/4 cup of batter for each pancake onto the griddle. Cook until golden brown on both sides. Serve hot.

<u>**Nutritional value**</u>

Carbs=17g

Protein=3g

Calories=129

Fat=4g

6.Yummy Veggie Omelet

Prep Time: 10 mins
Cook Time: 10 mins
Total Time: 20 mins
Servings: 2

Ingredients

- 2 tablespoons butter, divided
- 1 small onion, chopped
- 1 green bell pepper, chopped
- ¾ teaspoon salt, divided
- 4 large eggs
- 2 tablespoons milk
- ⅛ teaspoon freshly ground black pepper
- 2 ounces shredded Swiss cheese

Directions

1. Melt 1 tablespoon of butter in a medium skillet over medium heat. Cook onion and bell pepper in the butter until tender, about 4 to 5 minutes. Transfer to a bowl, season with 1/4 teaspoon of salt, and set aside.

2. In another bowl, beat eggs, milk, 1/2 teaspoon of salt, and pepper together.

3. Melt the remaining 1 tablespoon of butter in the skillet over medium heat. When bubbly, pour in the egg mixture and cook without stirring for about 1 minute until the bottom starts to set. Lift the edges with a spatula to let uncooked egg flow underneath. Continue cooking for 1 to 2 minutes until the centre starts to dry.

4. Sprinkle cheese over the omelette, add the vegetable mixture to one half, and fold the omelette over the vegetables with a spatula. Cook for about 1 minute until the cheese melts. Slide onto a plate, cut in half, and serve.

<u>Nutritional value</u>
Carbs=12g
Protein=22g
Calories= 398
Fat=34g

7.Southwest Breakfast Burritos

Prep Time:50 mins

Cook Time:15 mins

Total Time:1 hr 5 mins

Servings:20

Ingredients

- 12 large eggs
- ⅔ cup milk
- ½ teaspoon salt
- 2 tablespoons butter
- 1 pound bulk pork sausage
- 2 tablespoons minced garlic
- ½ red onion, diced
- 1 tomato, diced
- ¼ cup chopped fresh cilantro
- 1 (3.5 ounce) can diced jalapeños (Optional)
- 1 (1 ounce) package taco seasoning
- 1 ½ cups shredded Cheddar cheese
- 20 (6 inch) flour tortillas

Directions

1. Gather all ingredients.

2. In a large bowl, whisk eggs, milk, and salt. Heat butter in a large skillet over medium-high heat. Pour in the egg mixture and cook, stirring, until set, about 5 minutes.

3. Break up the cooked eggs into small pieces and place in a large bowl.

4. In the same skillet over medium heat, cook sausage and garlic for 5 minutes. Add onion and cook until the sausage is browned and crumbly. Drain excess grease.

5. Add the sausage mixture to the eggs. Stir in tomato, cilantro, jalapeños, and taco seasoning. Let cool to room temperature, then mix in Cheddar cheese.

6. Place a tortilla on your work surface. Spoon some filling onto the lower half of the tortilla. Shape the filling into a rectangle. Fold the bottom of the tortilla over the filling, then fold in the sides, and roll up tightly. Repeat with the remaining tortillas and filling.

7. Wrap each burrito in plastic wrap and freeze until ready to serve.

8. To serve, microwave burritos for 3 to 4 minutes until hot.

<u>Nutritional value</u>
Carbs=19g
Protein=12g
Calories=312
Fat=19g

8.Blueberry Smoothie Bowl

Prep Time:10 mins

Total Time:10 mins

Servings:1

Ingredients

<u>Smoothie:</u>

- 1 cup frozen blueberries
- ½ banana
- 2 tablespoons water
- 1 tablespoon cashew butter
- 1 teaspoon vanilla extract

<u>Toppings:</u>

- ½ banana, sliced
- 1 tablespoon sliced almonds
- 1 tablespoon unsweetened shredded coconut

Directions

1. Blend blueberries, half a banana, water, cashew butter, and vanilla extract until smooth. Pour into a bowl.

2. Top the smoothie with sliced banana, almonds, and coconut.

<u>Nutritional value</u>

Carbs=58g

Protein=5g

Calories=370

Fat=17g

9. Hearty Breakfast Muffins

Prep Time: 20 mins

Cook Time: 20 mins

Additional Time: 10 mins

Total Time: 50 mins

Servings: 12

Ingredients

- 2 carrots, shredded
- 2 bananas, mashed
- 1 zucchini, shredded
- ¼ cup vegetable oil
- ¼ cup yoghourt
- 2 eggs
- 1 cup whole wheat flour
- 1 ½ teaspoons baking soda
- ½ cup packed brown sugar
- ½ cup rolled oats
- ½ cup shredded coconut
- ½ cup chopped pecans
- ½ cup dried cherries
- 1 teaspoon ground cinnamon
- 1 teaspoon salt
- ½ teaspoon ground ginger

Directions

1. Preheat the oven to 375°F (190°C). Grease 12 muffin cups or line them with paper liners.

2. In a large bowl, mix together carrots, banana, zucchini, vegetable oil, yogurt, and eggs until well combined.

3. In another bowl, whisk together flour and baking soda. Add brown sugar, oats, coconut, pecans, cherries, cinnamon, salt, and ginger, stirring until coated in flour. Combine the banana mixture with the flour mixture until just mixed. Fill the muffin cups 2/3 full with the batter.

4. Bake for 18 to 22 minutes, until the tops spring back when lightly pressed. Cool in the tin for 10 minutes, then transfer to a wire rack to cool completely.

<u>Nutritional value</u>
Carbs=32g
Protein=4g
Calories=238
Fat=10g

10.Chocolate-Coconut Chia Pudding.

Prep Time:5 mins

Additional Time:1 hr

Total Time:1 hr 5 mins

Servings:3

Ingredients

- 1 cup almond milk
- ¼ cup chia seeds
- ¼ cup coconut flakes
- 1 tablespoon unsweetened cocoa powder
- 1 tablespoon white sugar
- ½ teaspoon vanilla extract
- 1 medium banana, sliced

Directions

1. In a bowl, combine almond milk, chia seeds, coconut flakes, cocoa powder, sugar, and vanilla extract. Mix well. Cover and refrigerate for 1 hour. Top with banana or your choice of fruit.

<u>Nutritional value</u>

Carbs=24g

Protein=4g

Calories=181

Fat=8g

Creative Alternatives to Traditional Breakfast Foods

1.Quinoa Porridge: Say goodbye to oats and hello to quinoa! This ancient grain is not only packed with protein and nutrients but also naturally free of galactose. Cook it up with your favourite plant-based milk, add a touch of honey or maple syrup, and top with fresh fruit and nuts for a hearty and wholesome breakfast.

2.Chia Seed Pudding: Chia seeds are a nutritional powerhouse and a fantastic alternative to dairy-based breakfasts. Simply mix chia seeds with your choice of plant-based milk and let it sit overnight to thicken into a creamy pudding-like consistency. Top with berries, sliced almonds, and a drizzle of agave syrup for a delightful morning treat.

3.Avocado Toast: Avocado toast has become a breakfast staple for good reason – it's delicious, nutritious, and incredibly versatile. Spread ripe avocado on whole grain toast and customise with toppings like sliced tomatoes, red pepper flakes, or a sprinkle of sea salt. It's a simple yet satisfying way to start your day on a healthy note.

4.Sweet Potato Hash: Who says breakfast has to be sweet? Swap out traditional breakfast potatoes for nutrient-rich sweet potatoes in this savoury hash. Simply dice sweet potatoes and sauté with onions, bell peppers, and your favourite seasonings until golden brown and crispy. Top with a poached egg or serve alongside scrambled tofu for a filling morning meal.

5.Coconut Yogurt Parfait: For those missing out on dairy yoghourt, coconut yoghourt is a fantastic alternative that's both creamy and delicious. Layer coconut yoghurt with fresh berries, granola, and a drizzle of honey or agave syrup for a breakfast parfait that's as beautiful as it is tasty.

6.Banana Pancakes: Who needs milk and eggs when you have bananas? These two-ingredient pancakes are a game-changer for anyone managing galactosemia. Simply mash ripe bananas and mix with flour to create a thick batter. Cook on a hot griddle until golden brown on both sides, then serve with your favourite toppings like sliced bananas, berries, or a dollop of almond butter.

7.Tofu Scramble: Say hello to your new favourite breakfast scramble! Tofu is a versatile ingredient that can be seasoned and cooked to perfection, mimicking the texture of scrambled eggs without the dairy. Sauté tofu with onions, peppers, spinach, and your favourite spices for a savoury and satisfying breakfast option.

8.Smoothie Bowl: Blend up a nutritious smoothie using your favourite fruits, leafy greens, and plant-based milk, then pour it into a bowl and top with crunchy granola, coconut flakes, and a drizzle of honey or agave syrup. It's a refreshing and energising way to kickstart your day without any dairy in sight.

Chapter:5

Lunchtime Favourites

1.Caribbean Chicken Salad

Prep Time:30 mins

Cook Time:15 mins

Additional Time:2 hrs

Total Time:2 hrs 45 mins

Servings:4

Ingredients

- 2 skinless, boneless chicken breast halves
- ½ cup teriyaki marinade sauce
- 2 tomatoes, seeded and chopped
- ½ cup chopped onion
- 2 teaspoons minced jalapeño pepper
- 2 teaspoons chopped fresh cilantro
- ¼ cup Dijon mustard
- ¼ cup honey
- 1 ½ tablespoons white sugar
- 1 tablespoon vegetable oil
- 1 ½ tablespoons cider vinegar
- 1 ½ teaspoons lime juice
- ¾ pound mixed salad greens
- 1 (8 ounce) can pineapple chunks, drained
- 4 cups corn tortilla chips

Directions

1. Put chicken in a bowl and cover it with teriyaki marinade sauce. Let it marinate in the fridge for at least 2 hours.

2. Mix tomatoes, onion, jalapeño pepper, and cilantro in a small bowl for salsa. Cover and refrigerate.

3. Prepare dressing by mixing mustard, honey, sugar, oil, vinegar, and lime juice in a small bowl. Cover and refrigerate.

4. Heat the grill on high.

5. Lightly oil the grill grate. Grill chicken for 6 to 8 minutes on each side until cooked through.

6. Place mixed salad greens on plates. Top with salsa, pineapple chunks, tortilla chips, and grilled chicken strips. Drizzle with dressing and serve.

<u>**Nutritional value**</u>

Carbs=70g

Protein=18g

Calories=475

Fat=12g

2.Easy Quinoa Salad

Prep Time:20 mins

Cook Time:15 mins

Total Time:35 mins

Servings:6

Ingredients

- 2 cups water
- 1 cup quinoa
- ¼ cup extra-virgin olive oil
- 2 limes, juiced
- 2 teaspoons ground cumin
- 1 teaspoon salt
- ½ teaspoon red pepper flakes, or more to taste
- 1 ½ cups halved cherry tomatoes
- 1 (15 ounce) can black beans, drained and rinsed
- 5 green onions, finely chopped
- ¼ cup chopped fresh cilantro
- salt and ground black pepper to taste

Directions

1. Boil water and quinoa in a saucepan, then simmer until quinoa is cooked and water is absorbed. Let it cool.

2. While quinoa cools, whisk olive oil, lime juice, cumin, salt, and red pepper flakes in a small bowl.

3. In a large bowl, combine quinoa, tomatoes, black beans, and green onions. Pour dressing over the mixture and toss to coat. Add cilantro and season with salt and pepper.

4. Serve right away or chill the salad in the fridge.

55

<u>Nutritional value</u>
Carbs=29g
Protein=8g
Calories=285
Fat=13g

3. Turkey Avocado Panini

Prep Time:17 mins
Cook Time:8 mins
Total Time:25 mins
Servings:2

Ingredients

- ½ ripe avocado
- ¼ cup mayonnaise
- 2 ciabatta rolls
- 1 tablespoon olive oil, divided
- 2 slices provolone cheese
- 1 cup whole fresh spinach leaves, divided
- ¼ pound thinly sliced mesquite smoked turkey breast
- 2 roasted red peppers, sliced into strips

Directions

1. Mash the avocado and mayonnaise together in a bowl until well combined.

2. Preheat a panini sandwich press.

3. Prepare the sandwiches by splitting the ciabatta rolls in half horizontally. Brush the bottom of each roll with olive oil. Place the bottoms of the rolls on the panini press, oil side down. Layer provolone cheese, spinach leaves, turkey breast, and roasted red pepper on each sandwich. Spread avocado mixture on the cut surface of each top, then place the top of the roll on the sandwich. Brush the top of the roll with olive oil.

4. Close the panini press and cook until the bun is toasted, with golden brown grill marks, and the cheese is melted, about 5 to 8 minutes.

<u>**Nutritional value**</u>

Carbs=42g

Protein=23g

Calories=725

Fat=53g

4.Sweet Potato, Carrot, Apple, and Red Lentil Soup.

Prep Time:25 mins

Cook Time:55 mins

Total Time:1 hr 20 mins

Servings:6

Ingredients

- ¼ cup butter
- 2 large sweet potatoes, peeled and chopped
- 3 large carrots, peeled and chopped
- 1 apple - peeled, cored, and chopped
- 1 onion, chopped
- ½ cup red lentils
- 1 teaspoon salt
- ½ teaspoon minced fresh ginger
- ½ teaspoon ground black pepper
- ½ teaspoon ground cumin
- ½ teaspoon chilli powder
- ½ teaspoon paprika
- 4 cups vegetable broth

Directions

1. In a large pot, melt butter over medium-high heat. Add sweet potatoes, carrots, apple, and onion. Cook and stir until onion is translucent, about 10 minutes.

2. Stir in lentils, salt, ginger, pepper, cumin, chili powder, and paprika. Pour in broth. Bring to a boil over high heat, then reduce to medium-low, cover, and simmer until lentils and vegetables are soft, about 30 minutes.

3. Use an immersion blender to purée the soup in the pot until smooth. Increase heat to medium-high and simmer for about 10 minutes until heated through. Add water as needed to reach your desired consistency.

<u>Nutritional value</u>
Carbs=55g
Protein=9g
Calories=324g
Fat=8g

5.Watermelon Caprese Appetisers

Prep Time:30 mins

Total Time:30 mins

Servings:4

Ingredients

- 3 sprigs fresh basil, stems removed
- 1 small watermelon, fruit removed with a melon baller
- 1 (8 ounce) package fresh mozzarella cheese, cut into small pieces
- 2 tablespoons olive oil
- 2 tablespoons balsamic vinegar
- salt and ground black pepper to taste

Directions

1. Cut basil leaves into 1-inch circles.

2. Alternate threading watermelon, mozzarella cheese, and basil leaves onto toothpicks. Arrange on a plate.

3. Drizzle olive oil and balsamic vinegar over toothpicks. Sprinkle with salt and black pepper.

Nutritional value

Carbs=28g

Protein=14g

Calories=345

Fat=20g

6.Mediterranean Zucchini and Chickpea Salad

Prep Time:25 mins

Total Time:25 mins

Servings:6

Ingredients
- 2 cups diced zucchini
- 1 (15 ounce) can chickpeas, drained and rinsed
- 1 cup halved grape tomatoes
- ¾ cup chopped red bell pepper
- ½ cup chopped sweet onion ½ cup crumbled feta cheese
- ½ cup chopped Kalamata olives
- ⅓ cup olive oil
- ⅓ cup packed fresh basil leaves, roughly chopped
- ¼ cup white balsamic vinegar
- 1 tablespoon chopped fresh rosemary
- 1 tablespoon capers, drained and chopped
- 1 clove garlic, minced
- ½ teaspoon dried Greek oregano
- 1 pinch crushed red pepper flakes (Optional)
- salt and ground black pepper to taste

Directions

1. Combine zucchini, chickpeas, tomatoes, red bell pepper, onion, feta cheese, Kalamata olives, olive oil, basil, vinegar, rosemary, capers, garlic, oregano, red pepper flakes, salt, and black pepper in a large bowl.

<u>**Nutritional value**</u>

Carbs=25

Protein=6g

Calories=279

Fat=19g

8. Black Bean and Corn Quesadillas

Prep Time:10 mins

Cook Time:30 mins

Total Time:40 mins

Servings:8

Ingredients

- 2 teaspoons olive oil
- 3 tablespoons finely chopped onion
- 1 (15.5 ounce) can black beans, drained and rinsed
- 1 (10 ounce) can whole kernel corn, drained
- ¼ cup salsa
- 1 tablespoon brown sugar
- ¼ teaspoon red pepper flakes
- 2 tablespoons butter, or as needed
- 8 (8 inch) flour tortillas
- 1 ½ cups shredded Monterey Jack cheese

Directions

1. Heat olive oil in a large saucepan over medium heat. Cook onion until softened, about 2 minutes. Add beans, corn, salsa, brown sugar, and red pepper flakes. Cook until heated through, about 3 minutes. Remove from heat.

2. Melt butter in a large skillet over medium heat. Place a tortilla in the skillet and sprinkle with Monterey Jack cheese and bean mixture. Top with another tortilla. Cook until golden on one side, then flip and cook until golden on the other side. Repeat with remaining tortillas and filling.

<u>**Nutritional value**</u>

Carbs=47g

Protein=15g

Calories=365

Fat=59

<u>**Strategies for Balanced Nutrition.**</u>

Balanced nutrition is not about deprivation or strict rules. It's about embracing a variety of flavours, colours, and nutrients to nourish both body and soul. Picture your plate as a canvas, ready to be adorned with a spectrum of vibrant hues and textures. From crisp greens to juicy fruits, from hearty grains to lean proteins, each element plays a vital role in achieving harmony.

Start your culinary adventure by exploring the produce aisle. Here, nature's bounty awaits, offering an array of fresh fruits and vegetables bursting with flavour and nutrients. Embrace the rainbow, opting for a diverse selection of colourful produce to ensure a broad spectrum of vitamins, minerals, and antioxidants. Whether it's leafy greens like spinach and kale or vibrant peppers and berries, each bite is a celebration of vitality.

Next, let's journey to the heart of the kitchen: the pantry. Here, we find a treasure trove of grains, legumes, nuts, and seeds, each offering a unique blend of fibre, protein, and essential fats. Whole grains like quinoa, brown rice, and oats provide sustained energy and a wealth of nutrients, while legumes such as lentils and chickpeas add a hearty dose of plant-based protein. Don't forget the nuts and seeds, rich in heart-healthy fats and micronutrients, perfect for adding crunch and flavour to any dish.

Now, let's talk about the star of the show: protein. Whether you're a meat lover or a plant-based enthusiast, there are plenty of options to satisfy your cravings while supporting your health goals. Lean meats like chicken, turkey, and fish are excellent sources of protein, while also providing essential vitamins and minerals. For those following a plant-based diet, tofu, tempeh, and legumes offer a delicious alternative, packed with protein and flavour.

Of course, no meal is complete without a touch of indulgence. Here, moderation is key as we savour the sweetness of life. Opt for natural sweeteners like honey, maple syrup, or dates, which not only add sweetness but also bring depth and complexity to your dishes. And let's not forget about fats, essential for flavour and satiety. Choose heart-healthy fats like olive oil, avocado, and nuts, and use them sparingly to enhance the taste and texture of your creations.

Easy-to-Pack Meals for On-the-Go.

When it comes to crafting meals for life on the move, simplicity is key. As a seasoned professional chef, I understand the need for easy-to-pack meals that don't sacrifice flavour or nutrition. Whether you're heading out for a day of adventure or simply need a quick bite between meetings, these recipes are designed to keep you fueled and satisfied no matter where your day takes you.

Let's start with breakfast, the most important meal of the day. Instead of reaching for sugary cereals or greasy fast food, why not try making your own breakfast burritos? Simply scramble some eggs, sauté some veggies like bell peppers and onions, and add a sprinkle of cheese. Roll it all up in a whole wheat tortilla, wrap it in foil, and you've got a portable breakfast that's packed with protein and flavour.

For lunch, think beyond the sandwich. One of my favourite on-the-go meals is a quinoa salad with roasted vegetables. Cook up a batch of quinoa according to the package instructions, then toss it with some roasted veggies like cherry tomatoes, zucchini, and bell peppers. Drizzle with a simple vinaigrette made from olive oil, balsamic vinegar, and a squeeze of lemon juice, and you've got a light and refreshing meal that's perfect for eating on the run.

When it comes to snacks, homemade energy bars are a game-changer. Forget the store-bought versions loaded with artificial ingredients and preservatives – these homemade bars are made with wholesome ingredients like oats, nuts, and dried fruit. Mix everything together in a bowl, press it into a baking dish, and bake until golden brown. Once cooled, cut into bars and wrap individually for a quick and easy snack that will keep you going throughout the day.

Dinner doesn't have to be complicated, even when you're away from home. One-pot meals are a lifesaver when you're on the go, and my go-to is a simple pasta primavera. Cook up some whole wheat pasta until al dente, then toss it with sautéed veggies like broccoli, carrots, and peas. Finish with a drizzle of olive oil and a sprinkle of Parmesan cheese, and dinner is served.

Of course, no meal is complete without a sweet treat to satisfy your cravings. Instead of reaching for store-bought cookies or candy bars, why not make your own trail mix? Simply combine your favourite nuts, seeds, and dried fruit in a resealable bag, and you've got a portable snack that's perfect for satisfying your sweet tooth on the go.

Chapter:6

Dinner Delicacies

---

1. Grilled salmon

Prep Time:10 mins

Cook Time:15 mins

Additional Time:2 hrs

Total Time:2 hrs 25 mins

Servings:6

Ingredients

- 1 ½ pounds salmon fillets
- lemon pepper to taste
- garlic powder to taste
- salt to taste
- ⅓ cup soy sauce
- ⅓ cup brown sugar
- ⅓ cup water
- ¼ cup vegetable oil

Directions

1. Season salmon fillets with lemon pepper, garlic powder, and salt.

2. Mix soy sauce, brown sugar, water, and vegetable oil until sugar dissolves. Put salmon in a resealable bag, add soy sauce mixture, seal, and coat fish. Refrigerate for at least 2 hours.

3. Preheat grill to medium heat and lightly oil the grate.

4. Grill salmon, discarding marinade, until fish flakes easily with a fork, about 6 to 8 minutes per side.

<u>Nutritional value</u>
Carbs=14g
Protein=22g
Calories=320
Fat=25g

2. Beef Wellington

Prep Time:30 mins

Cook Time:40 mins

Total Time:1 hr 10 mins

Servings:8

Ingredients

- 2 ½ pounds beef tenderloin
- 4 tablespoons butter, softened, divided
- 2 tablespoons butter
- 1 onion, chopped
- ½ cup sliced fresh mushrooms
- 2 ounces liver paté
- salt and pepper to taste
- 1 (17.5 ounce) package frozen puff pastry, thawed
- 1 large egg yolk, beaten
- 1 (10.5 ounce) can beef broth
- 2 tablespoons red wine

Directions

1. Preheat the oven to 425°F (220°C).

2. Put beef tenderloin in a baking dish and spread 2 tablespoons of softened butter over it.

3. Bake until browned, about 10 to 15 minutes. Remove beef from the pan and keep pan juices aside. Let the beef cool.

4. Increase oven temperature to 450°F (230°C).

5. Melt 2 tablespoons butter in a skillet over medium heat. Cook onion and mushrooms for 5 minutes. Remove from heat and let cool.

6. Mix paté and remaining 2 tablespoons of softened butter in a bowl; season with salt and pepper. Spread paté mixture over beef. Top with onion and mushroom mixture.

7. Roll out puff pastry dough to 1/4-inch thickness and place beef in the centre.

8. Fold and seal all edges, ensuring seams aren't too thick. Put beef in a 9x13-inch baking dish, cut slits in the dough, and brush with egg yolk.

9. Bake for 10 minutes. Reduce heat to 425°F (220°C) and continue baking until pastry is golden brown, about 10 to 15 minutes. The thermometer should read between 122 to 130°F (50 to 54°C) for medium rare. Let it rest.

10. Heat reserved pan juices in a small saucepan over high heat. Stir in beef broth and red wine; boil until slightly reduced, about 5 minutes. Strain and serve with beef.

11. Serve hot and enjoy!

<u>Nutritional value</u>
Carbs=30g
Protein=28g
Calories=744
Fat=58g

3. Lobster risotto

Prep Time:15 mins

Cook Time:1 hr

Total Time:1 hr

Servings:6

Ingredients

- ¼ cup olive oil, divided
- 2 onions, chopped
- 6 cups chicken broth
- 1 shallot, chopped
- 1 clove garlic, chopped
- 1 ½ cups Arborio rice
- ½ cup white wine
- 1 tablespoon honey
- 3 tablespoons butter
- 1 cup light cream
- 1 tablespoon paprika
- 1 teaspoon cayenne pepper
- ¼ cup sherry
- 2 cups cooked lobster meat
- ½ cup shredded Parmesan cheese
- 1 pinch salt and ground black pepper to taste

Directions

1. Heat 2 tablespoons of oil in a large skillet over medium heat. Cook onions until very tender, about 20 minutes.

2. Bring chicken broth to a boil in a pot, then reduce heat to low to keep it simmering.

3. Heat remaining 2 tablespoons of oil in a large, flat-bottom pan over medium-high heat. Cook shallot and garlic until fragrant, about 2 minutes. Add Arborio rice and cook until it begins to brown, about 3 minutes. Pour in wine and cook for 1 minute.

4. Stir 1 cup of chicken broth into rice mixture and cook until absorbed, stirring constantly. Repeat adding broth, 1 cup at a time, until all broth is used, stirring constantly until absorbed each time, about 30 minutes.

5. Stir honey into onions and cook for 5 more minutes.

6. Stir butter into rice mixture until melted. Add cream and stir until mixture thickens, about 3 minutes. Add paprika, cayenne pepper, and sherry; mix well. Add lobster meat and cook until heated through, about 3 minutes. Mix in Parmesan cheese until melted. Add onion mixture and mix well. Season with salt and pepper.

<u>Nutritional value</u>
Carbs=60g
Protein=19g
Calories=565
Fat=25g

4. Chicken Marsala

Prep Time: 10 mins

Cook Time: 20 mins

Total Time: 30 mins

Servings: 4

Ingredients

- ¼ cup all-purpose flour for coating
- ½ teaspoon salt
- ¼ teaspoon ground black pepper
- ½ teaspoon dried oregano
- 4 medium skinless, boneless chicken breast halves - pounded 1/4 inch thick
- 4 tablespoons butter
- 4 tablespoons olive oil
- 1 cup sliced mushrooms
- ½ cup Marsala wine
- ¼ cup cooking sherry

Directions

1. Gather all ingredients.

2. In a shallow dish or bowl, combine flour, salt, pepper, and oregano.

3. Coat chicken pieces in the flour mixture.

4. In a large skillet, melt butter in olive oil over medium heat. Add chicken and lightly brown.

5. Turn chicken pieces over and add mushrooms. Pour in wine and sherry.

6. Cover skillet and simmer chicken for 10 minutes, turning once, until cooked through and juices run clear.7. Serve and enjoy!

5. Vegetable stir-fry with tofu

Prep Time:30 mins

Cook Time:15 mins

Total Time:45 mins

Servings:4

Ingredients

- 1 tablespoon vegetable oil
- ½ medium onion, sliced
- 1 tablespoon fresh ginger root, finely chopped
- 2 cloves garlic, finely chopped
- 1 (16 ounce) package tofu, drained and cut into cubes
- 1 cup baby corn, drained and cut into pieces
- 1 green bell pepper, seeded and cut into strips
- 1 carrot, peeled and sliced
- 1 small head bok choy, chopped
- 2 cups fresh mushrooms, chopped
- 1 ¼ cups bean sprouts
- 1 cup bamboo shoots, drained and chopped
- ½ teaspoon crushed red pepper

Sauce:

- ½ cup water
- ¼ cup rice wine vinegar
- 2 tablespoons honey
- 2 tablespoons soy sauce
- 2 tablespoons water
- 2 teaspoons cornstarch

Garnish:

- 2 medium green onions, thinly sliced diagonally

Directions

1. Heat oil in a large skillet over medium-high heat. Cook onion for 1 minute. Add ginger and garlic; cook for 30 seconds. Add tofu and cook until golden brown.

2. Add corn, bell pepper, and carrot; cook for 2 minutes. Stir in bok choy, mushrooms, bean sprouts, bamboo shoots, and crushed red pepper. Cook until heated through, then remove from heat.

3. Make sauce: Combine water, vinegar, honey, and soy sauce in a small saucepan. Simmer for 2 minutes. Mix water and cornstarch in a small bowl; add to vinegar mixture. Simmer until the sauce thickens.

4. Pour sauce over tofu-vegetable mixture. Garnish with green onions.

Cooking Techniques and Flavor Enhancers.

When it comes to cooking for someone with galactosemia, it's essential to understand the condition and how certain cooking techniques and flavour enhancers can make a big difference. Galactosemia is a rare genetic metabolic disorder where the body is unable to metabolise galactose properly, a sugar found in milk and dairy products. This means individuals with galactosemia need to avoid these foods and ingredients containing galactose.

I've encountered various dietary restrictions, but galactosemia presents unique challenges. However, with the right approach, it's possible to create delicious and satisfying meals that adhere to these restrictions without sacrificing flavour.

One of the key cooking techniques to master when cooking for someone with galactosemia is substitution. Since dairy products are off the table, it's important to find suitable alternatives that provide similar textures and flavours. For example, coconut milk can be used as a substitute for cow's milk in recipes like creamy soups and sauces. Its rich and creamy consistency adds depth to dishes without the use of dairy.

Another important technique is to focus on fresh, whole ingredients. By using fresh fruits, vegetables, herbs, and spices, you can elevate the flavour of your dishes without relying on dairy or processed ingredients. Experimenting with different herbs and spices allows you to create unique flavour profiles that will tantalise the taste buds.

In addition to substitution and fresh ingredients, cooking methods also play a crucial role in flavour enhancement for individuals with galactosemia. Techniques such as roasting, grilling, and sautéing can help to caramelise the natural sugars in foods, intensifying their flavour without the need for dairy-based ingredients. These cooking methods also add depth and complexity to dishes, making them more satisfying and enjoyable.

When it comes to flavour enhancers, herbs and spices are your best friends. Ingredients like garlic, ginger, turmeric, cumin, and paprika can add a burst of flavour to any dish without the need for dairy. Fresh herbs like basil, cilantro, parsley, and mint can also brighten up a dish and provide a refreshing contrast.

Another flavour enhancer to consider is acid. Ingredients like lemon juice, lime juice, vinegar, and citrus zest can add a tangy brightness to dishes, balancing out rich flavours and adding depth. Additionally, using umami-rich ingredients like mushrooms, tomatoes, soy sauce, and nutritional yeast can help to create a savoury, satisfying taste experience.

Chapter:7

Snack Attack

---

1. Microwave Popcorn

Prep Time:2 mins
Cook Time:3 mins
Total Time:5 mins
Servings:3

Ingredients

- ½ cup unpopped popcorn
- 1 teaspoon vegetable oil
- ½ teaspoon salt, or to taste

Directions

1. Gather all the ingredients.

2. Mix unpopped popcorn and oil in a cup or small bowl.

3. Put the coated corn into a brown paper lunch sack, and sprinkle with salt. Fold the top of the bag over twice to seal.

4. Microwave at full power for 2 1/2 to 3 minutes, or until there are pauses of about 2 seconds between pops. Open the bag carefully to avoid steam, and pour into a serving bowl.

5. Enjoy your popcorn!

2.Veggie Stroganoff

Prep Time:10 mins

Cook Time:18 mins

Total Time:28 mins

Servings:4

Ingredients

- 3 tablespoons Spectrum Naturals Canola Oil, divided
- 1 medium onion, chopped
- 1 large clove garlic, minced
- 1 (8 ounce) package sliced button or cremini mushrooms
- 1 (170 gram) package Yves Veggie Cuisine® Beef Veggie Tenders
- 2 tablespoons all-purpose flour
- 1 cup Imagine Organic Vegetable Broth
- 1 teaspoon Dijon mustard
- ½ teaspoon ground thyme
- ½ teaspoon seasoning salt
- ½ cup The Greek Gods™ Traditional Plain Yogurt or sour cream
- 1 tablespoon chopped fresh parsley
- 1 (8 ounce) package Egg or egg-free noodles, cooked according to package directions

Directions

1. Heat 1 tablespoon of oil in a large non-stick skillet over medium heat. Add onion and cook for 6 minutes until soft. Add garlic and mushrooms; cook for 2 minutes, stirring often.

2. Add Beef Veggie Tenders and cook for 1 minute. Transfer everything to a large plate.

3. Add remaining 2 tablespoons of oil to the skillet. Stir in flour and cook for about 2 minutes until lightly browned.

4. Mix in broth, Dijon, thyme, and seasoning salt. Cook for 2 minutes until thickened. Return mixture to skillet. Cover and simmer over low heat for 5 minutes.

5. Stir in yoghourt and warm through. Sprinkle with parsley and serve over hot cooked noodles.

3.Barley Salad With Almonds And Apricots

Prep Time:1 hr 25 mins

Total Time:1 hr 25 mins

Servings:11

Ingredients

- 1 ½ cups pearl barley
- 4 ½ cups water
- 1 tablespoon canola oil
- 1 red onion, thinly sliced
- ¾ cup dried apricots, sliced
- ½ cup sliced almonds
- 2 tablespoons chopped fresh parsley
- 1 cup plain low-fat yoghourt
- 2 tablespoons honey
- 1 lemon, juiced
- ½ teaspoon ground cinnamon
- ½ teaspoon ground turmeric
- ½ teaspoon salt
- 1 pinch ground nutmeg

Directions

1. Rinse barley, then cook in boiling water until tender, about 45 to 50 minutes. Let it cool.

2. Sauté onion in oil until golden brown.

3. Combine barley, onion, apricots, almonds, and parsley in a serving dish.

4. Mix yoghourt, honey, lemon juice, cinnamon, turmeric, salt, and nutmeg in a small bowl. Pour over barley mixture and toss. Serve at room temperature.

4.10-Minute Rice Cakes

Prep Time: 5 mins

Cook Time: 5 mins

Total Time: 10 mins

Servings: 1.

Ingredients

- ½ cup cooked white rice
- 1 egg
- 1 tablespoon chopped fresh basil (Optional)
- 1 teaspoon milk
- salt and ground black pepper to taste
- 1 ½ teaspoons butter

Directions

1. Combine rice, egg, basil, milk, salt, and pepper in a bowl.

2. Melt butter in a skillet over medium heat. Divide rice mixture into two equal portions and cook until browned on one side, about 3 minutes. Flip and cook until browned on the other side, about 2 more minutes.

5. Apple Peanut Butter Cake.

Prep Time:30 mins

Cook Time:40 mins

Additional Time:5 mins

Total Time:30 mins

Servings:16

Ingredients

- Reynolds® Parchment Paper
- ¾ cup all-purpose flour
- ¼ cup whole wheat flour
- 1 teaspoon baking powder
- ½ teaspoon ground cinnamon
- ¼ teaspoon salt
- ⅛ teaspoon ground allspice
- ¾ cup packed brown sugar
- 2 tablespoons butter, softened
- 1 egg
- ¼ cup applesauce
- ½ teaspoon vanilla
- ¾ cup tart apple, such as Granny Smith, peeled and diced
- ¼ cup peanut butter chips

<u>Peanut Butter Glaze:</u>

- 3 tablespoons creamy peanut butter
- 2 tablespoons milk, or more as needed

Directions

1. Preheat the oven to 350°F. Line an 8x8-inch baking pan with Reynolds® Parchment Paper.

2. In a medium bowl, whisk together all-purpose flour, whole wheat flour, baking powder, cinnamon, salt, and allspice. Set aside.

3. In another medium bowl, cream together sugar and butter with an electric mixer until light and fluffy. Add egg and beat until combined. Mix in applesauce and vanilla. Gradually add the flour mixture on low speed. Stir in chopped apple and peanut butter pieces. Spread the batter into the prepared pan.

4. Bake for 35 to 40 minutes or until a toothpick inserted into the center comes out clean.

5. Let the cake cool in the pan for 5 minutes, then lift it out using the parchment paper and transfer it to a wire rack to cool completely. Transfer the cake to a cutting board using the parchment paper.

6. Drizzle the Peanut Butter Glaze over the cooled cake and let it stand until the glaze sets before slicing.

7. For the Peanut Butter Glaze: In a small bowl, stir together powdered sugar, creamy peanut butter, and milk until it reaches a thick drizzling consistency.

Portion Control and Mindful Eating Tips.

First and foremost, let's talk about portion control. With galactosemia, managing the intake of galactose, a sugar found in dairy products, is crucial. One effective approach is to visualise portion sizes using everyday objects. For example, a serving of meat should be about the size of a deck of cards, while a serving of pasta should be around the size of a tennis ball. This simple trick can help you gauge your portions without the need for measuring cups or scales.

Next, let's discuss mindful eating. Mindful eating is about paying attention to the sensory experience of eating, including the taste, texture, and aroma of food. For individuals with galactosemia, it's essential to focus on foods that are low in lactose or lactose-free alternatives. Incorporating a variety of nutrient-dense foods such as fruits, vegetables, whole grains, and lean proteins can help ensure a well-rounded diet while minimising the risk of galactose buildup.

When planning your meals, consider incorporating smaller, more frequent meals throughout the day to maintain steady energy levels and prevent overeating. Additionally, be mindful of your hunger cues and strive to eat slowly, savouring each bite. This not only enhances the dining experience but also allows your body to recognize when it's comfortably full, reducing the likelihood of overindulgence.

In addition to portion control and mindful eating, it's important to be mindful of hidden sources of galactose in processed foods. Always read food labels carefully and opt for products labelled as lactose-free or galactose-free whenever possible. Cooking from scratch using fresh, whole ingredients is not only a great way to avoid hidden sources of galactose but also allows you to customise recipes to suit your dietary needs and preferences.

When it comes to cooking, simple swaps can make a world of difference. For example, replace cow's milk with lactose-free alternatives such as almond milk, coconut milk, or soy milk in recipes calling for milk. Similarly, swap out regular yoghourt for lactose-free yoghurts or dairy-free alternatives like coconut yoghurt or almond yoghurt. These substitutions not only accommodate your dietary restrictions but also add unique flavours and textures to your dishes.

Celebrating Special Occasions with Delicious Sweets

When it comes to celebrating, nothing brings people together quite like a decadent dessert. Whether it's a birthday, anniversary, or holiday gathering, the right sweet treat has the power to elevate any occasion from ordinary to extraordinary. From rich chocolate cakes to delicate pastries filled with luscious creams, each dessert has its own story to tell.

One of the most rewarding aspects of being a pastry chef is witnessing the joy that my creations bring to others. There's something truly magical about seeing the delight on someone's face as they take that first bite of a perfectly crafted dessert. It's a moment that never fails to warm my heart and remind me why I chose this path.

But creating memorable desserts isn't just about taste – it's also about presentation. A beautifully plated dessert not only looks stunning but also adds to the overall dining experience. Whether it's a simple garnish of fresh berries or an intricate sugar sculpture, attention to detail is key in creating a masterpiece that will leave a lasting impression.

Of course, no celebration would be complete without the perfect cake. From towering wedding cakes adorned with intricate designs to whimsical birthday cakes that capture the spirit of the occasion, the possibilities are endless. As a chef, I take pride in customising each cake to reflect the unique personalities and preferences of my clients, ensuring that every bite is as unforgettable as the moment itself.

But it's not just about the big events – everyday moments deserve to be celebrated too. Whether it's a quiet evening at home or a casual get-together with friends, there's always an excuse to indulge in something sweet. From simple cookies and brownies to elegant tarts and mousses, there's no shortage of options when it comes to satisfying your sweet tooth.

I'm constantly inspired by the endless variety of flavours and textures that can be found in the world of desserts. From classic combinations like chocolate and peanut butter to more exotic pairings like mango and coconut, there's always something new to explore and experiment with. And while I may have spent years honing my skills, I'm always learning and discovering new techniques to push the boundaries of what's possible in the world of pastry.

But perhaps the greatest joy of all is sharing my love of desserts with others. Whether it's teaching a cooking class, hosting a dessert tasting event, or simply sharing a slice of cake with a friend, there's nothing quite like the connection that is forged over a shared love of food. In a world that can often feel divided, desserts have a unique ability to bring people together, transcending cultural barriers and fostering a sense of unity and joy.

So whether you're celebrating a milestone moment or simply savouring the sweetness of everyday life, remember to indulge in the simple pleasure of a delicious dessert. After all, life is too short to deny yourself the simple joys that can be found in a perfectly crafted sweet treat. As a seasoned professional chef, I can attest that there's no greater satisfaction than seeing the smiles of delight that my desserts bring to those I serve. So go ahead, treat yourself – you deserve it.

<u>Baking Tips and Tricks for Success.</u>

<u>1.Start with Quality Ingredients:</u> Just like a masterpiece painting starts with high-quality paints, a delicious baked good begins with the best ingredients. Always opt for fresh, high-quality ingredients for superior taste and texture.

<u>2.Measure Accurately:</u> Baking is a science, and precise measurements are crucial. Invest in a good set of measuring cups and spoons, and always follow recipes carefully, levelling off ingredients for accuracy.

<u>3.Preheat Your Oven:</u> Before you even think about mixing ingredients, preheat your oven. This ensures that your baked goods start cooking at the right temperature from the get-go, leading to even baking and perfect results.

<u>4.Use Room Temperature Ingredients:</u>
Unless specified otherwise, most recipes call for ingredients like eggs, butter, and milk to be at room temperature. This allows them to blend seamlessly into the batter, creating a smoother texture.

<u>5.Don't Overmix:</u> While it's tempting to keep mixing until every last lump is gone, overmixing can lead to tough, dense baked goods. Mix ingredients until just combined for the best results.

<u>6.Invest in Quality Tools:</u> A good set of baking pans, mixing bowls, and utensils can make a world of difference in your baking endeavours. Look for sturdy, durable tools that will stand the test of time.

7.Learn the Power of Leavening Agents: Baking powder and baking soda are your secret weapons when it comes to achieving the perfect rise in your baked goods. Understand how they work and how to adjust them to suit different recipes.

8.Don't Peek: It's tempting to open the oven door to check on your creations, but resist the urge. Every time you open the door, you let out valuable heat, which can affect the baking process. Trust your oven and use a timer instead.

9.Rotate Your Pans: Ovens can have hot spots, leading to uneven baking. To combat this, rotate your pans halfway through the baking time to ensure that everything bakes evenly.

10.Let it Cool: Patience is key when it comes to baking. Allow your baked goods to cool completely before diving in. This allows flavours to develop and textures to set, resulting in a more delicious end product.

11.Practice Makes Perfect: Like any skill, baking takes practice. Don't be discouraged if your first attempt isn't perfect. Keep experimenting, learning, and improving with each bake.

12.Get Creative: While it's important to master the basics, don't be afraid to get creative and put your own spin on classic recipes. Add different flavours, textures, and

decorations to make your baked goods truly unique.

Chapter:8

Beyond the Kitchen

Living Well with Galactosemia.

In this book, I'll share with you my insights, tips, and recipes tailored specifically for those living with galactosemia, a rare genetic disorder that affects the body's ability to process galactose, a sugar found in milk and dairy products.

Understanding Galactosemia:

Before we delve into the culinary delights, let's take a moment to understand galactosemia. It's a condition where the body lacks the enzyme needed to break down galactose, leading to potential complications if not managed properly. This means avoiding foods containing lactose, the sugar found in dairy products, which can be challenging but not impossible.

The Importance of Diet:

A well-balanced diet is essential for everyone, but it's especially crucial for those with galactosemia. By choosing the right foods and ingredients, you can maintain optimal health and minimise the risk of complications. Throughout this book, I'll show you how to create flavorful meals that are not only safe but also satisfying and nutritious.

Navigating the Grocery Store:

One of the first steps in living well with galactosemia is knowing what to look for at the grocery store. Stock up on fresh fruits and vegetables, whole grains, lean proteins, and dairy alternatives such as soy, almond, or coconut milk. Read labels carefully, avoiding products that contain lactose or hidden sources of galactose.

Cooking with Confidence:

Cooking should be a joyful experience, not a source of stress. With a few simple swaps and substitutions, you can transform any recipe into a galactosemia-friendly masterpiece. Experiment with new flavours and ingredients, and don't be afraid to get creative in the kitchen.

Recipe Makeovers:

Many classic recipes can be modified to suit a galactosemia-friendly diet. From creamy pasta dishes to decadent desserts, I'll show you how to recreate your favourite meals without sacrificing taste or texture. Get ready to impress your friends and family with dishes that are as delicious as they are nutritious.

Meal Planning Made Easy:

Planning ahead is key to success when living with galactosemia. Take some time each week to map out your meals, making sure to include a variety of flavours and nutrients. Batch cooking can also be a lifesaver, allowing you to prepare large quantities of food in advance and freeze for later use.

Eating Out:

Eating out can be a challenge when you have dietary restrictions, but it's not impossible. Look for restaurants that offer dairy-free options or are willing to accommodate special requests. And don't be afraid to speak up – most chefs are more than happy to customise dishes to meet your needs.

The Power of Community:

Living with galactosemia can feel isolating at times, but you're not alone. Seek out support groups and online communities where you can connect with others who understand what you're going through. Share recipes, swap tips, and lend a listening ear – together, we can thrive.

In conclusion, navigating the culinary landscape with galactosemia requires creativity, patience, and a deep understanding of suitable ingredients and cooking techniques. The journey towards mastering a galactosemia-friendly diet begins with education and experimentation. Through this cookbook, beginners are equipped with essential knowledge about galactosemia, empowering them to take control of their health and well-being without sacrificing the joy of cooking and eating.

With the recipes provided, beginners can embark on a flavorful adventure, discovering new ingredients and innovative cooking methods tailored to their dietary needs. From breakfast delights to savoury dinners and tempting desserts, this cookbook offers a diverse array of dishes that are not only delicious but also safe for individuals with galactosemia.

Moreover, the cookbook emphasises the importance of mindful ingredient selection and label reading, enabling readers to make informed choices when shopping for groceries. By adopting a proactive approach to meal planning and preparation, beginners can confidently navigate social gatherings and dining out experiences while adhering to their dietary restrictions.

Beyond the kitchen, this cookbook fosters a sense of community among individuals living with galactosemia. Through shared experiences and culinary tips, beginners can connect with others facing similar challenges, finding inspiration and support along their journey towards better health.

In essence, the Galactosemia Cookbook for Beginners serves as a comprehensive guide and companion for individuals newly diagnosed with galactosemia. It empowers them to embrace their dietary restrictions with optimism and creativity, transforming mealtimes into moments of culinary delight and nourishment. With each recipe crafted with care and consideration, this cookbook invites beginners to embark on a flavorful adventure towards a healthier and happier life.

BONUS PAGE

1.30 DAY MEAL PLAN

Day 1:
Breakfast: Oatmeal with almond milk and fresh fruit.
Lunch: Grilled chicken salad with mixed greens, vegetables, and vinaigrette dressing.
Dinner: Baked salmon with quinoa and steamed broccoli.

Day 2:
Breakfast: Smoothie made with coconut milk, spinach, banana, and protein powder.
Lunch: Turkey wrap with lettuce, tomato, and avocado on a gluten-free tortilla.
Dinner: Stir-fried tofu with vegetables and brown rice.

Day 3:
Breakfast: Chia seed pudding made with rice milk and topped with berries.
Lunch: Lentil soup with gluten-free bread.
Dinner: Grilled shrimp skewers with roasted sweet potatoes and green beans.

Continue to vary meals throughout the month, ensuring they are free from dairy products and high-galactose foods. Incorporate plenty of fruits, vegetables, lean proteins, and alternative dairy products such as almond milk, coconut milk, or rice milk. Always read labels carefully to avoid hidden sources of galactose. It's also essential to consult with a registered dietitian or healthcare provider for personalised guidance and meal planning.

2.SMART INGREDIENTS SWAP.

Part 1: Understanding Smart Swaps
Before we dive into the world of ingredient swaps, let's first understand why they're so important. Smart ingredient swaps allow us to cut down on unhealthy fats, sugars, and processed ingredients, while boosting nutrition and flavour. By making strategic substitutions, we can create dishes that are not only delicious but also better for our bodies.

Part 2: The Power of Herbs and Spices
Herbs and spices are the secret weapons in any chef's arsenal, adding depth, complexity, and flavour to dishes. Instead of relying on salt and unhealthy seasonings, experiment with fresh herbs like basil, cilantro, and rosemary, or spice things up with cumin, paprika, and turmeric. These simple swaps will take your dishes from ordinary to extraordinary.

Part 3: Healthier Fats for Cooking
Fat is an essential component of cooking, but not all fats are created equal. Instead of reaching for butter or vegetable oil, consider using healthier alternatives like olive oil, avocado oil, or coconut oil. These fats are rich in monounsaturated and polyunsaturated fats, which can help lower cholesterol and reduce the risk of heart disease.

Part 4: Whole Grains for Satisfying Meals
Swap out refined grains like white rice and pasta for nutrient-rich whole grains like quinoa, brown rice, and whole wheat pasta. Not only do whole grains provide more fibre, vitamins, and minerals, but they also have a nuttier flavour and chewier texture that adds depth to your dishes. Try incorporating whole grains into your favourite recipes for a healthier twist.

Part5:Sneaky Vegetable Substitutions
Vegetables are nature's gift to chefs, offering a rainbow of colours, flavours, and nutrients to play with. Get creative with your vegetable substitutions by swapping out traditional ingredients with nutrient-packed alternatives. For example, use zucchini noodles instead of pasta, cauliflower rice instead of white rice, or mashed sweet potatoes

instead of mashed potatoes. These simple swaps will add extra vitamins and minerals to your meals while cutting down on carbs and calories.

Part 6: Sweet Treats without the Guilt

Who says you can't enjoy sweet treats while eating healthy? With smart ingredient swaps, you can indulge in your favourite desserts guilt-free. Replace refined sugars with natural sweeteners like honey, maple syrup, or dates, and swap out white flour for almond flour or oat flour. You'll be amazed at how delicious and satisfying healthy desserts can be.

Congratulations! You've now mastered the art of smart ingredient swaps, unlocking a world of culinary possibilities. By making simple substitutions in your cooking, you can create dishes that are not only delicious but also nutritious and satisfying. So go ahead, experiment with different ingredients, and let your creativity run wild in the kitchen. Your taste buds—and your body—will thank you for it. ***Happy cooking!***

3.THE SMART SHOPPER'S GUIDE TO DECODING FOOD LABELS.

1.Ingredients List: Think of the ingredients list as your culinary compass, guiding you through the maze of additives and preservatives. Pay attention to the first few ingredients, as they make up the bulk of the product. Look for recognizable, whole foods like fruits, vegetables, and whole grains. Beware of lengthy lists filled with unpronounceable chemicals – if you can't pronounce it, do you really want to eat it?

2.Nutrition Facts: Don't be fooled by flashy claims on the front of the package – the real story lies in the nutrition facts panel. Keep an eye on serving sizes, as they can be deceiving. Compare the calories, fat, sugar, and sodium content to similar products to make an informed choice. Remember, just because something is labelled as "low-fat" or "sugar-free" doesn't necessarily mean it's healthy.

3.Allergen Warnings: For those with food allergies or intolerances, allergen warnings are crucial. Scan the label for common allergens like nuts, dairy, eggs, and gluten. Manufacturers are required by law to clearly label these ingredients, but it's always better to be safe than sorry. If you're unsure, reach out to the manufacturer for clarification.

4.Certifications and Seals: Keep an eye out for certifications and seals of approval from reputable organisations like the USDA Organic, Non-GMO Project, and Certified Gluten-Free. These labels indicate that the product has met certain standards and undergone rigorous testing. While they're not foolproof, they can help steer you towards healthier, more sustainable options.

5.Marketing Buzzwords: Beware of marketing buzzwords designed to lure you in with promises of health and wellness. Terms like "natural," "artisanal," and "wholesome" are vague and unregulated, meaning they can be slapped on just about anything. Instead, focus on the facts – what's actually in the product and how it fits into your overall diet.

6.Expiration Dates: Don't overlook expiration dates – they're there for a reason. Pay attention to both "sell by" and "use by" dates, and never consume food that's past its prime. When in doubt, trust your senses – if something smells off or looks questionable, it's better to be safe than sorry.

7.Country of Origin: Knowing where your food comes from can provide valuable insight into its quality and safety. Look for labels indicating the country of origin, especially when it comes to fresh produce, meat, and seafood. Whenever possible, opt for locally sourced products to support your community and reduce your carbon footprint.

8.Packaging and Sustainability: Finally, consider the environmental impact of your food choices. Opt for products with minimal packaging and eco-friendly materials whenever possible. Look for recycling symbols and choose products that prioritise sustainability and waste reduction.

By arming yourself with knowledge and a discerning eye, you can navigate the world of food labels with confidence and clarity. Remember, the choices you make at the grocery store have a profound impact on your health, your wallet, and the planet. So take your time, read the labels, and choose wisely. Happy shopping!

4.FOOD LIST ENCYCLOPEDIA.

Let's start with the basics. In the produce section, you'll find an array of fruits and vegetables bursting with flavour and nutrients. From crisp apples to juicy tomatoes, each item is described in detail, including tips on selecting, storing, and preparing them to perfection. Whether you're a novice cook or a seasoned pro, you'll find plenty of inspiration in these pages to elevate your dishes to new heights.

Next up, we explore the world of grains and legumes. From rice and quinoa to lentils and chickpeas, these staples form the foundation of many cuisines around the globe. Learn about different varieties, their flavour profiles, and cooking methods to add depth and texture to your meals. With a little creativity, you can turn these humble ingredients into culinary masterpieces that will impress even the most discerning palate.

No food encyclopaedia would be complete without a section dedicated to proteins. From succulent cuts of meat to tender seafood, there's something here to satisfy every appetite. Discover the difference between grass-fed beef and grain-fed beef, or learn how to properly fillet a fish for a perfectly cooked seafood dish. With detailed instructions and insider tips, you'll become a protein pro in no time.

Of course, no meal is complete without a touch of flavour, which is why we've included a comprehensive guide to herbs, spices, and condiments. From aromatic basil to fiery chilli peppers, each ingredient adds its own unique flair to dishes, transforming them from ordinary to extraordinary. Learn how to balance flavours, experiment with different combinations, and unleash your inner chef with confidence.

But our exploration doesn't stop there. The Food List Encyclopedia also delves into the world of dairy and alternative dairy products, offering insights into the various types of milk, cheese, and yoghourt available on the market today. Whether you're lactose intolerant or simply looking to expand your culinary horizons, you'll find plenty of options to suit your needs and preferences.

And let's not forget about sweets and treats. Indulge your sweet tooth with a decadent array of desserts, from classic cakes and cookies to innovative creations that push the boundaries of taste and texture. With step-by-step recipes and helpful hints, you'll be whipping up delectable delights in no time, impressing friends and family alike with your newfound baking prowess.

In addition to individual ingredients, the Food List Encyclopedia also explores various cooking techniques, from grilling and roasting to sautéing and steaming. Each method is explained in detail, with tips on when and how to use them to achieve the best results. Whether you're a fan of slow cooking or prefer to whip up quick and easy meals, you'll find plenty of inspiration to suit your style.